# The Science Of Yoga

By
Meenakshi Swamy
Translated by
Neelam Sharma
Illustrated by
Surendra Suman

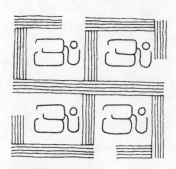

Children's Book Trust, New Delhi

*Vyaktitwa-Vikas Aur Yog* won the First Prize in the category Non-fiction/Information in the Competition for Writers of Children's Books in Hindi. *The Science of Yoga* is rendered from the original.

Text typeset in 12/16 pt. Times New Roman

EDITED BY GEETA MENON

ISBN 81-7011-934-0

Published by Children's Book Trust, Nehru House, 4 Bahadur Shah Zafar Marg, New Delhi-110002 and printed at its Indraprastha Press. Ph: 23316970-74 Fax: 23721090 e-mail: cbtnd@vsnl.com Website: www.childrensbooktrust.com

# Foreword

Yoga is a technique for allround development of man including his physical, mental, intellectual, emotional and spiritual aspects.

It is sad that people are not fully aware of the science of yoga, in spite of it being an invaluable boon of Indian culture. People harbour misconceptions about this science. Some people think yoga means but physical exercises; some others believe it is leading life as an ascetic; and still others think that it is a means of performing miracles. In reality, yoga is much more than all these.

The book is an attempt to remove misconceptions and to explain the meaning of yoga, which involves eight steps, namely—*yama, niyama,* asana, *pranayama, pratyahara, dharana, dhyana* and *samadhi,* in a simple and lucid manner.

Usually the books on yoga, which are readily available, are meant for adults. They impart knowledge about the asanas. One needs to take great care while performing the asanas, and should initially perform them under the guidance of an expert. The effort here throws light on the scientific relevance of yoga and a yogic lifestyle.

The book describes how a person can develop his personality by regular practice of yoga. The precautions one should take while practising yoga are important.

The book will help to re-establish cultural values, some important ones being *brahmacharya* (celibacy) and love for all living beings.

One can learn the scientific technique of yoga through this book. Regular practice will help youngsters to be rid of many of their problems such as dejection, mental conflict, tension on account of career, presence of negative tendencies in the character, aggressive temperament, lack of power of discrimination, loss of intellectual and mental faculties, wayward habits, and so on.

Whereas many people relate yoga to a particular religion, yoga is related to the entire human race.

Today, when the influence of yoga and its vogue is increasing in the West, it has become necessary for us to acquaint the future generations of India with its scientific technique.

It is believed that the book will attract children towards yoga and increase their knowledge about this discipline. This is a prime need for a society being increasingly subjected to tension and violence.

Positively the literature will encourage one to adopt a yogic lifestyle.

The writing attempted is in a simple style. Citing examples that relate to the interests and problems of children, it seeks to clarify their doubts to arouse their interest.

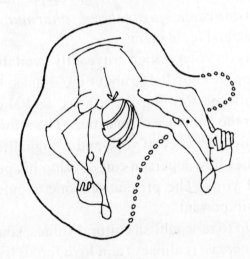

# Introductory

You must have at some time seen a piece of wood floating on the ocean. It is tossed and toyed with, by the waves; despite its desire to reach the shore, it cannot do so. If the waves so wish, they can throw the piece onto the bank.

Your condition is very similar. You are like a toy in the hands of nature. You desire to make a mark in the world, yet find it difficult to make that possible.

With the regular practice of yoga, you transform yourself into an expert swimmer. When you attain that skill, you are no longer at the mercy of the waves. You can cut your way through them to reach the shore. That is, you achieve your goal through your own endeavour.

With the help of yoga, you can do many jobs successfully. You can excel in studies, sports, dance and drama and can be a good orator. More, you can lend a helping hand to your mother and guide your younger brothers and sisters in their studies.

At present you may desire to do all these, but are unable to do so. When you sit down to study, you start having a backache, you get tired while writing or you develop a headache owing to strain in your eyes. So you give up studies and go to play. After some time you start panting, get tired for want of concentration in your game and you get defeated easily. You may try to do some other work, you fail to put your heart into it.

Given a chance to deliver a speech, you feel nervous, shaky and are unable to speak. Many among you are so scared that you fall ill with approaching examinations.

You have to work very hard for all that you wish to achieve, and this requires enormous energy and strength.

While preparing for a play, you manage to work hard but when you step on the stage you forget your dialogues. In the examination hall, you find that you have forgotten the answers to the questions that you had crammed thoroughly well earlier. Your mind becomes totally blank.

It is possible that you are overtaken by jealousy when you see your friend has obtained the first position in the examination. You do not like his success and try to run him down whenever you get the opportunity. If you happen to secure the first position yourself, you become so vain that you do not speak to anybody, study less and think too high of yourself, with the result that you come down the ladder of success.

You get angry at being admonished by your mother or teacher or when you are unable to get an exercise book from your friend. Sometimes you fly into a rage and talk senselessly to others spoiling the good relationship you had. You pick up a fight when angry and if your friend is weaker than you, you become violent and at times you let your anger out on your siblings or on your servants. If your inability thwarts you, then you scheme against your friend. With the result, you start breathing heavily; your heartbeat increases and sometimes you even tremble in anger. All this wastes a good deal of your time. It ruins your health and self-control. Many a time you commit blunders which lead to serious consequences. At times impertinence follows.

Sometimes you are depressed at losing a trivial thing, be it a pencil or an eraser and cannot put your heart into any work. You may have noticed that in extreme cases, some students who fail in the examination become so sad and depressed that they commit suicide.

At times you are lured by your friend into doing some kind of mischief like plucking guavas or *jamuns* from somebody's garden. He takes you along with him and if the gardener arrives, he flees, leaving you behind. Now you are caught and beaten up. You think the worst of your friend. The truth remains that it was not only your friend's mistake but yours too. Your friend had invited you but it was your weak mind that had accepted his offer. You may have initially refused his offer but you were half-hearted; your weak mind gave in ultimately.

If you had restrained your mind and not followed your friend, no harm would have come to you but you did not possess enough strength to control your mind. A weak mind wanders here and there.

Our mind is endowed with great strength but loses all because of its aimless wanderings. While sitting in the class and listening to your teacher, your mind roams in the playground. You think of playing well and winning. Your mind switches over to the comics you had read a day earlier and you fantasize about becoming a superman. Within a short time, your mind is distracted; you think of films.

Meanwhile, you are not listening to your teacher and do not understand what he has explained. Sensing your absent-mindedness, your teacher asks you about what is being taught. You are taken unawares and are unable to answer him.

Why? It happens because your mind was restless. Even though you were physically present in the class, you were thinking of the playground, comics or films! As a result, you were unable to concentrate on what was being taught.

The same thoughts haunt you at home also and you are unable to study. When you bring a bad report card home, you are admonished by your parents and this spoils your chances of visiting a hill station, going on tours, watching films or reading comics in the summer vacations. Instead, you have to study your course books!

Look, how your fragile mind has spoilt everything! If you were attentive in class and had listened to the teacher, everything would have been all right. Sad! your weak mind does not allow you to concentrate on your work. Its goalless drifting creates difficulties and problems for you.

If you are talking to your friend while cycling or are absorbed in some other thoughts, do you know what might happen? An accident! Since you are not concentrating on your cycling, you will remain unaware of the approaching vehicle or its blaring horns. The result could be disastrous. If you ride your bicycle with attention and apply the brakes at the right time, you will reach your destination safe and early.

You must have seen a horse-rider. If the rider knows how to control the reins, he can go to any place; but if he lacks control, it is the horse who will lead him and not vice versa. The horse can even throw him down and cause him serious injury.

Your mind too acts in a similar fashion. If you have the ability to control your mind and train it to act on your command, you can be very successful.

The mind contains immense strength but cannot use it because much of it is spent in aimless wanderings. If you apply the entire energy in one direction and with purpose, you can surely make a mark in the world.

You must have seen a monkey in a zoo or in its natural habitat. It loves jumping from tree to tree, branch to branch, plucking fruits and throwing them half-eaten and destroying things.

The mind too behaves like a monkey, maybe worse! You might have noticed how disciplined the monkey becomes when under the control of a trainer it performs many tricks. If you wish, you can discipline your mind the way a trainer does a monkey.

You will be able to study at the time you are supposed to study, and play at the time you are supposed to play. Given full devotion, attention and concentration, you will achieve success.

## A Lifestyle

Is it possible to direct the entire energy of your restless mind to a particular direction?

Yes, it is possible through yoga. If you adopt yoga as your lifestyle, many things will become easy for you. This can be done by making yoga a part of your life. For instance, you bathe, eat and play everyday; similarly, you should practise yoga daily. If you eat, sleep, and live according to the rules of yoga, it will become your lifestyle.

Yoga will heal your body first. For doing any work successfully you need a healthy body. Thereafter, restlessness and ·fickleness of the mind will gradually disappear. You will acquire the power of concentration and your intellect and memory will improve. You will excel in studies as well as in sports. You will be successful in performing dance, drama and music and can win laurels for your oratorial skills.

Do you know what yoga is?

8

You must have heard about yoga and watched it on TV. You might think that yoga is various kinds of exercises or that it is a method of treatment of diseases.

Some of you may think that yoga means living like an ascetic and meditating in a forest or forsaking life.

Alternately, you may also think that yoga means performing miracles, such as walking on water, eating or walking on burning charcoal, eating glass, flying in the air or producing fruits, sweets, clothes or any other thing by a wave of the hand.

The truth is that yoga is not the science of *tantra-mantra* (mystical methods for attaining supernatural powers) and performing miracles. Again, physical exercises alone do not make yoga. Yoga has a higher meaning.

Yoga is a way of leading an ideal life. By following yoga we can have allround development of our mind, body and soul.

The regular practice of yoga helps in the physical, mental, intellectual and spiritual development of human beings. Yoga will create a healthy body and a healthy mind. These sustain noble thoughts.

The word 'yoga' is derived from the Sanskrit root *yuja* which means 'to unite the soul with the Supreme Soul of which we are a part'.

The goal of all humanity and all religion is to unite with the Supreme. Yoga makes it possible.

Much has been said about yoga by the sages. Patanjali has written in his *Yoga Sutra:*

*Yogashchitvrittinirodha*

(Yoga is the control of the mind.)

Yoga works as a check on this tendency of the mind. Checking the vague wanderings of the mind and directing it to useful tasks is yoga. Control over the mind means training it to act according to our wishes. Yoga is the reins of our mind.

You may be thinking what mind is. What does it look like?

Mind is a collection of thoughts. It is formless and cannot be seen. Whatever we think is the mind. Mind is action. Commanding the mind means controlling the thoughts.

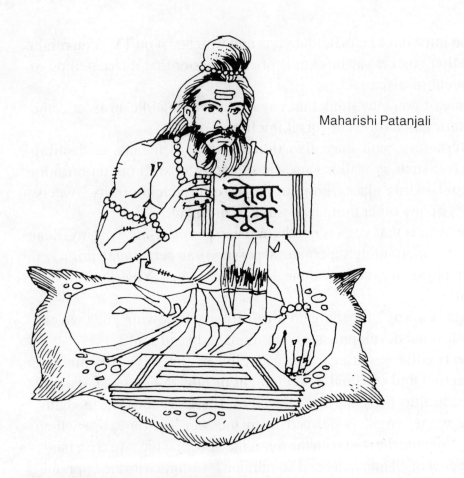
Maharishi Patanjali

The *Bhagavad Gita* says:

*Yogah karmasu kaushalam*

(Excellence in work is yoga.)

Excellence in work means doing any work efficiently. For performing any work well, we need to have a serene mind. As said earlier, with a serene mind you can do any work properly. If your mind is roaming while doing a particular job, you cannot hope to do it properly.

Yoga is a way of living which calms the mind and improves our ability too.

The *Gita* says:

*Samatvam yog uchyate*

(*Samabhava* or equilibrium of mind is yoga.)

*Sambhava* means to remain balanced in happiness as well as in sorrow. According to *Yoga Vasistha:*

*Manah prashamanopayah yog ityabhidheeyate*

(Yoga is the means of keeping the mind calm.)

The agitated mind creates problems like anger, tension and diseases. That is why it is essential to soothen the mind with the practice of yoga.

Swami Vivekananda said, "Yoga awakens the dormant Divinity that dwells in all of us." Man has duality of character. He has animal-like as

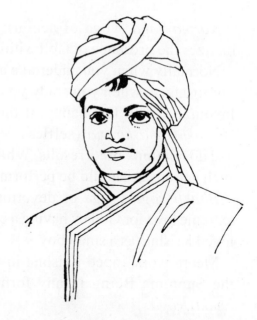

Swami Vivekananda

well as god-like instincts in him. Owing to the influence of animal instincts, he indulges in cruel, barbarous and violent actions. When he possesses divine qualities, he becomes loving, tender and sensitive towards all. Yoga curbs the violent feelings and makes us happy.

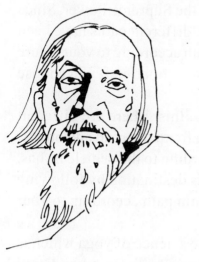

Sri Aurobindo

According to Sri Aurobindo, "Yoga is the process of allround development of man." Yoga helps in the complete development of an ideal personality. An ideal personality means physical, mental, intellectual, emotional and spiritual development.

## Paths Of Yoga

Yoga has many paths. The following four are the most significant:

*Karma yoga* (yoga of action): According to *karma yoga,* man realizes the presence of God within himself by doing selfless work.

Normally when you undertake a task, you first think of its reward. For instance, when you study you think of the result; if the result is favourable, you feel happy; if the result is bad, you feel unhappy. By *nishkama karma* (selfless service) you feel happy in action and do not think of its results. While pursuing this path, keep in mind such actions as should be performed for the good of all.

*Bhakti yoga* (yoga of devotion): In *bhakti yoga,* you develop extreme love for God by having a close relationship with Him. Surdas loved Krishna as a small boy.

Meera worshipped Krishna in the form of her husband. Loving the Supreme Being in any form of close relationship is called *bhakti yoga.*

*Gyana yoga* (yoga of knowledge): In *gyana yoga,* man feels the presence of the Supreme Form through knowledge, intellect and wisdom.

*Raja yoga* (king of yoga): As its name implies, it is the king of all yogas. According to this yoga, you have to exercise control over the mind, develop strong will power and by strictly following the prescribed path, you attain realization.

All paths lead to one destination, that is, the Supreme Power. Since human beings possess varied dispositions, different paths have been chalked out. You can choose a particular path according to your nature and can follow it. It is easier to reach your destination if you choose a path of your own.

It can be explained in a simple way like this. There are different paths for reaching a particular place, like a footpath, road and others. A person can choose a particular path according to the vehicle he has. If he does not possess any, he can reach his destination by following the footpath. Similarly, you choose a certain path according to your nature and capacity.

You will be very happy to know that the science of yoga which is essential for the development of the human body, mind and soul originated in India.

Yoga is the matchless and invaluable gift of our ancient Indian civilization. It is logical, and achieves its goal through gradualism. It is fully integrated. About 5,000 years ago, Maharishi Patanjali established the science of yoga.

Before Maharishi Patanjali, the knowledge related to yoga was scattered in the Upanishads, Vedas and other sacred texts. Patanjali collected all the relevant knowledge, compiled and systematized them.

For the allround development and benefit of mankind, Patanjali introduced the techniques of eight-fold yoga which he named as *Ashtanga yoga.*

Patanjali was a great scientist and an intellectual. You must have heard about Einstein. Where Einstein mastered the science of the physical world, Patanjali mastered the inner world of man.

There is a world existing inside man. Patanjali was the scientist of the inner world of man and he had a thorough knowledge of the inner world.

The whole world is grateful to India for its contribution to the science of yoga. And we are indebted to Maharishi Patanjali. He is celebrated for his contributions to the science of yoga, Sanskrit grammar and ayurveda.

We pay our homage to him in the prayer conducted before starting the practice of yoga:

*Yogen chittasya padenvacham*
*Malamshareerasya cha vedhyaken*
*Yopakaraatam pravaram muneenam*
*Patanjalim pranjjaliran tosmi*

(Patanjali's gifts to the human race are the science of yoga for removing mental vices, grammar for removing defects in the language and the science of ayurveda to remove physical disorders.)

Many people think that yoga is related to the Hindu religion. It is not so. Yoga is not related to any particular religion. Hindus have only discovered it.

Yoga is meant for mankind, to whatever religion, community, language or race the people may belong to. Anyone who has a body, mind, intellect and soul can practise yoga.

## A Universal Science

Yoga is useful in all places whether you are in India, America, France or Iran. You can practise it anywhere, in a village or in a city. You do not need any material or instrument. You just need a clean and well-ventilated place. You are required to take a balanced diet.

Yoga is based on certain principles. By performing a certain exercise you get a certain result. For example, adopting *yogasanas* will make the body flexible. By performing *pranayama* you will have control over your breathing. By practising a particular *asana* (sitting, meditating) you can avoid a particular disease.

Yoga, like all sciences, is experimental. The experiments are performed on the human body, mind and soul. Yoga is definitely a science because it is not simply based on belief but is based on the results derived from experimentation. As the principles of mathematics are proved true at all places and times, so are the principles of yoga.

Let us take an example. In arithmetic, two plus two is equal to four. This was correct many years ago; same as it is today. This will hold true in any corner of the world. The laws of yoga are similar. If years ago it was possible to control your breathing system (*pranayama*), today the same law holds good.

There are two types of actions in the world, the art of *bhoga* (enjoyment) and that of *tyaga* (renunciation).

Ability to enjoy life is an art. Everybody is not capable of enjoying the pleasures of life. To enjoy nutritious food is an art. To exercise check over the mind by taking only a limited quantity of food is an art of renunciation.

You do not know either the art of enjoyment or the art of abstinence. You take food in a hurry but are unable either to relish or digest it. Even if you find the food tasty you are not really able to enjoy it and gulp it down hastily. Although your tummy is full, you do not feel satisfied and eat more than what is required. If you learn to exercise restraint at the proper time, you will keep good health. Since you do not restrict yourself, you fall ill.

14

Yoga teaches you the art of enjoyment as well as the art of abstinence. It does not deter you from enjoying life but it is essential to stop at an appropriate time.

The regular practice of yoga will discipline your mind to the extent that you will know where to put an end to enjoyment and where to exercise restraint.

So, yoga is an art to create a healthy body and a serene mind.

Since this art is acquired by systematic technique and training, it is a science.

### Patanjali Sutra

Patanjali composed the *Patanjali Sutra* in four chapters and 196 *sutras* (formulae). The four chapters are *Samadhipada, Sadhanapada, Vibhutipada* and *Kaivalyapada.*

*Patanjali Sutra* is the science of *raja yoga*. By treading the path, you attain control over the mind and achieve determination.

By inculcating the eight-fold path of yoga in your life, you can make yoga your lifestyle. Then your personality will develop rapidly and you can progress in every field of life. The eight steps of yoga are described in the following *sutra:*

*Yamaniyamasanapranayamapratyaharadhãranãdhyana samadhayoashtavangaani*

*yama, niyama,* asana, *pranayama, pratyahara, dharana, dhyana, samadhi*—these eight steps are described below:

### Yama

*Yama* means non-violence, truth, non-stealing, celibacy and non-acceptance of help. By following these principles, the mind becomes pure.

*Ahimsasatyasteya brahmacharyaparigraha yamaah*

*Ahimsa* is non-violence. *Ahimsa* means not hurting anyone by your body, mind, speech and action. Have you experienced that whenever you intend hurting anybody you also suffer and even when you think ill of anybody, you feel perturbed yourself? You get spiritual contentment by cultivating the feeling of non-violence towards living beings.

*Satya* means truthfulness because what is real is the truth.

*Asteya* means not to steal. Stealing is not only stealing of objects but also of ideas or work done by others for one's own benefit.

*Brahmacharya* means celibacy, renunciation of all desires not only by the body but the mind and speech.

*Aparigraha* means non-acceptance of charity even in distress

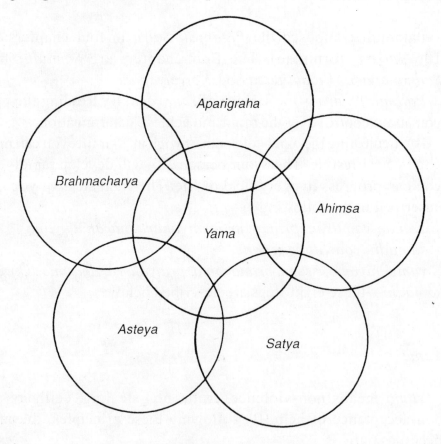

Parts of *Yama*

16

(what you have not earned). Even so, we should not hesitate to help others in need. When we help others we feel nice.

### Niyama

*Shaucha santosha tapah svadhyaya*
*ishwarapranidhanani niyamah*
(The practice of *shaucha, santosha, tapasya, svadhyaya* and *isvarapranidhana* is *niyama.*)

*Shaucha* means cleanliness of body. There are two types of *shaucha,* namely, external cleanliness and internal cleanliness.

External cleanliness includes keeping yourself clean by taking baths and so on. It also includes cleanliness of the various passages within the body through various methods like *kapalabhati, nauli, sankha prakshalana.*

It is easy for various diseases to attack the body if we do not keep it clean. By bathing and by cleaning our internal system, how fresh and active we feel! Lack of cleanliness makes us remain dirty, lazy and sick.

Internal cleanliness includes keeping your mind pure by following the truth and doing your duty. You have noticed that if you speak the truth and perform duties entrusted to you honestly, your mind gets immense solace; but if you lie, you are scared of being caught and then you have to face the consequences! In that state of mind, you are not able to perform your duties properly. You are always scared when you do not finish your homework, you cannot take interest in sports and are scared of being admonished by the teacher in class. If you have not studied throughout the year, how scared you feel at the time of the examination! However, if you have studied seriously throughout the year you need not fear at all. Thus, by treading the path of truth and by performing your duties honestly, which are a part of internal cleanliness, you can purify your mind.

This is the way to remain contented *(santosha)*. It is important.

Many people complain of drawbacks in their life and are, therefore,

17

not able to take advantage of what they have already got. On the other hand, a contented person always remains happy with whatever he has got.

*Tapasya* (austerities) means controlling the body by means of fasting, so on. Yoga lays emphasis on food. It is necessary to avoid food items which are tasty yet harmful to the body. Taking fried and oily food and meat makes the body fat and lazy letting it prone to diseases. If your body is unhealthy, you cannot do any work, for a healthy mind and a healthy body go together.

You are tempted by A, B, C, so on, and you eat them without temperance. Controlling such temptation is considered *tapasya*.

You should be careful about the type of food you eat because food has direct relevance to your body and mind. You can understand this better if you visit a zoo where you find that an elephant, despite being big in size, is calm by nature mainly because of the food that it eats, whereas the lion falls into the category of violent animals inasmuch as it is carnivorous. Food has the quality of creating gentleness or an aggressive nature.

Apart from the nature of food, you should also be careful about the quantity of food. Food should be consumed according to the requirement of the body, neither more nor less. Excessive food promotes sluggishness and increases fat in the body which invites a number of diseases. Taking food less than the required quantity is detrimental to health because this makes the body weak and slowly the mental and intellectual faculties of the body weaken.

The food consumed should be balanced, nutritious and proportionate to the needs of the body.

*Svadhyaya* means to study sacred texts which purify our mind and give us happiness. The Vedas and *Sastras* impart very important, useful and beneficial education to us which enrich our knowledge and sharpen our intellect. You have known that what we read influence our thinking. *Svadhyaya* includes chanting of *mantras*.

There are three ways of chanting mantras or *japa—vachika, upansu* and *manas*.

*Japa* (recitation) which is audible is called *vachika. Japa* which is

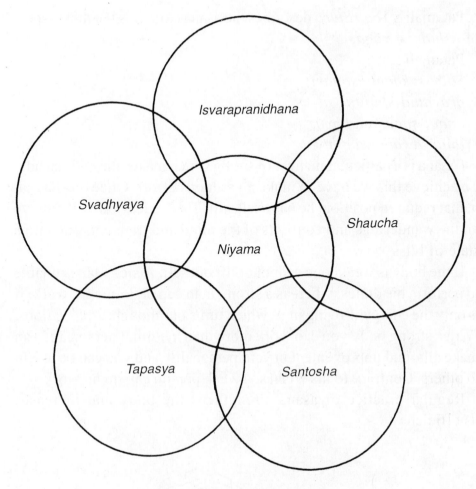

Parts of *Niyama*

not audible but where lip movement is evidently felt is called *upansu*, and the *japa* which we do in our mind concentrating on the meaning of the *mantra* is the best *japa*. It is called *manas japa*.

*Isvarapranidhana* means to praise, adore, remember, pray, worship and to please the particular form of the deity in which you have faith.

## Asana

It is a myth that asana and yoga are one and the same. In reality asana is only a part of yoga.

Patanjali's *Yoga Sutra* describes the asanas too. It is the third aspect of *ashtanga yoga*.

Patanjali says:

*Sthir sukham asanam*
*prayatna shaithilyat*
*anant samapatebhyas*
*tatau dwandwanbhiyat*

(Asana is a particular manner of sitting which makes the body steady. To achieve this we have to make an arduous effort. Once one has sat in that required position, he has to sit still. This endeavour will remove all the wanderings and conflicts of the mind and transport one into a state of bliss.)

If the body is weak, one cannot uplift oneself. A sick man is unable to perform his duties, whereas a strong man can do immense work. It is only the energy flowing in us which turns our thoughts into actions. With a strong body you can work more than a normal person and can make allround improvement in your personality and you can be useful to others. Contrary to his wishes, a weak person can do no work.

Regular practice of asana strengthens the body and increases its efficiency.

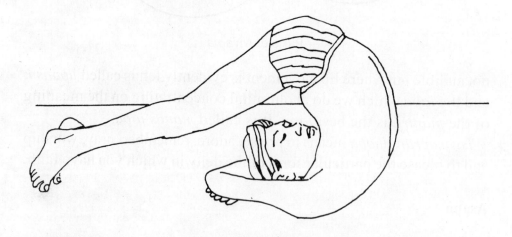

*Halasana* helps in digestion

The objective of asanas is to enhance the capabilities of the body to make maximum work possible.

After following the principles of *yama* (control) and *niyama* (rules) certain physical and mental *kriyas* (exercises) are required to be performed regularly. This will enable you to work at a stretch.

For example, while studying you are required to remain seated for a long time. You are unable to do so in spite of your best wishes because your body gives in and you develop a backache and stiffness in your shoulders. Asanas will help you to work at a stretch without hurting your body.

Asanas should be performed on a mat in a clean, well-ventilated and solitary place. It is not advisable to perform asanas in a polluted and noisy place.

Asanas should be performed early in the morning before sunrise or in the evening. They should always be performed on an empty stomach and never immediately after taking meals.

When you start with asanas, you find that your body does not have the required suppleness. In the beginning it is difficult to perform asanas perfectly. You are unable to turn and bend your body as you desire owing to the accumulation of fat in the joints. Therefore, a little physical exercise is necessary before performing asanas.

Sportsmen exercise before starting their games. They do so to acquire flexibility and to warm their body.

Physical exercises conducted before performing asanas include exercising your body, standing at one place and bending your knees, heels, elbows, toes and fingers, neck, spinal cord, so on.

These are called *sithilikarna* exercises and *gatisila asanas*. *Surya namaskara* is both a *sithilikarna* exercise and a *gatisila asana*. It removes the stiffness of the body and increases the rhythm of breathing. The nervous system gets stimulated. These exercises make the body so flexible for purpose of asanas.

The next step is *yogasana*. The *sthira* (stationary) asanas are done at a slow pace. While performing them you have to concentrate on your body.

After positioning your body in a particular posture, you let it remain *sthira* for some time.

These asanas provide rest to the nervous system. They help in the normal functioning of the heart and the lungs. The blood pressure also remains normal. Asanas remove mental tension and give peace of mind.

### Pranayama

According to Patanjali, sitting steadily in any asana and controlling the inhaling and exhaling process is *pranayama*.

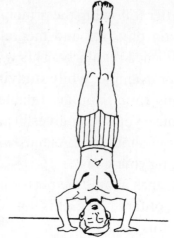

*Seershasana* enhances blood circulation

*Tasmin satishwas prashwasogati vichhedah pranayamah*
(Control over breathing is *pranayama*.)

It is the energy called *prana* which pervades the entire universe. All vibrating energies are *prana*. All material energies like heat, light, gravity, magnetism and electricity are *prana*.

This energy is present in all human beings alike, and indeed in all creations, sometimes in its dormant form and sometimes in its manifest form. Normally what we breathe in and breathe out is the *prana*, creating the rhythm of life.

*Prana* is not merely this but much more. The entire cosmos visible to us is actually the creation of *prana* and all actions are performed by this life force.

The Upanishads tell us that *prana* is the consciousness of life. *Prana* is considered equal to the soul. The life force which pervades all creatures of the universe such as an ant, an elephant, a sparrow, a fish, a frog and even a human being is the *prana*. They are born out of it, continue because of it and when they die, their *prana* merges with

22

the *prana* of the universe. Our life too is based on this life force.

Functions of the body are performed by the five types of *prana vayu:*

*Prana vayu*: It exists in the upper part of the body and controls the breathing process.

*Apana vayu*: It exists in the lower part of the body and controls the excretory as well as the reproductive system.

*Samana vayu*: It boosts the digestive process.

*Udana vayu*: This energy flows through the throat and controls the vocal cord.

*Vyana vayu*: This energy pervades the entire body. The energy that we get from food and from inhaling is carried by *vyana* to the arteries, veins and nerves.

*Prana* and mind are closely related. It is only through *pranayama* that we control our mind. When the *prana* is strong, the desires remain under control and, as a result, the mind becomes stable.

*Pranayama* is an art which, by means of different techniques, make breathing systematic and rhythmic.

## Stages

*Pranayama* has three stages:

*Puraka* (inhaling)—This stimulates the breathing process.

*Rechaka* (exhaling)—It expels the impure air and toxic matter out of the body; and

*Kumbhaka*—It is the process of retaining the breath for some time and also carrying the energy to the various parts of the body.

*Kumbhaka* is of three types: *Antah kumbhaka* is to retain the breath inside; *bahya kumbhaka* is to exhale but not inhale; and *keval kumbhaka* is the process which implies neither inhaling nor exhaling.

*Pranayama* disciplines the breathing process and improves health. You become enthusiastic and optimistic in attending to all work. Thoughts, actions and desires are streamlined properly. It makes your life balanced and will power strong. One could exercise self-control by *pranayama.*

People generally believe that the breathing process goes on automatically and that they do not have any control over it. In reality, through perseverance and different techniques of yoga, we can train it so much that it can follow our dictates.

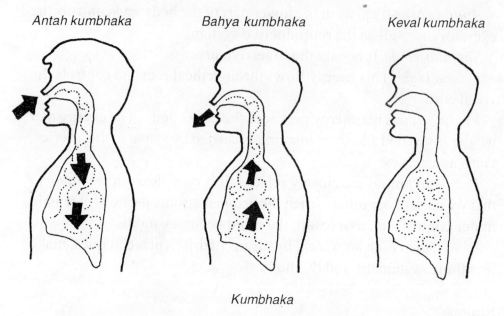

Antah kumbhaka  Bahya kumbhaka  Keval kumbhaka

Kumbhaka

Controlling the breathing process in this way is *pranayama*.

The existence of life in the body depends upon the movement of the lungs. When this movement stops, all activities of the body cease. Some persons train their bodies in such a manner that even after the movement of the lungs stop, other activities of the body continue.

You must have seen, heard or read about such yogis who remain buried under the ground and stop breathing for many days yet remain alive. This is possible by training their bodies through the techniques of *pranayama*.

Many of us are not aware of the right way of breathing and that is the reason our bodies remain weak and we fall a victim to different diseases. *Pranayama* regulates the faulty system of breathing and corrects it. It purifies the body, mind and intellect.

Mastery over *pranayama* opens the gateway of immense power. As has been stated earlier, all the cosmic forces of the universe are

24

manifested in the *prana*. So, for those who have controlled *prana*, the entire physical and mental forces become easily accessible.

You know that there are several nerve centres in our body and the sensation from one nerve centre to the other is carried by a maze of 72,000 nerves. Among these, embedded in the spinal cord are two important nerves, the *ida* and the *pingala*. In the marrow of the spine runs the *sushumna*, a dormant channel.

It is believed that at the base of the *sushumna* rests the *kundalini* which is a dormant power. It is awakened by *pranayama* and then it starts travelling upwards through the *sushumna*. As it travels upwards, it unfolds several *chakras* (centres of power) one by one. Thus a person practising yoga undergoes transcendental experiences and acquires supernatural powers. When *kundalini* reaches the head, man attains supreme knowledge.

You must have learnt about the power of electrons. When all the electrons move in one direction it is known as electric motion. If in a room all the electrons are made to move in one direction the room will be transformed into a powerful battery.

Similarly, when the breathing system is brought into rhythm and is regulated, all the electrons of the body travel in one direction. Then the restless mind moves in a single direction and achieves strong will power. It acquires speed and power, like that of electricity.

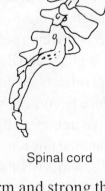

Spinal cord

When the *prana* is disciplined, it becomes so firm and strong that merely by its vibration, it can heal others physically and mentally.

You must have heard that merely by the sight or touch of the sages, people are healed of ailments of body and mind and become healthy. By practising *pranayama* the sages strengthen their *prana* so much that they can heal merely by the vibrations emanating from their bodies.

According to *yoga sastra,* the first step is to control the function of the lungs. Many activities continue in our body but we are unable to perceive them as our mind tends to wander outside. When the same mind turns inward then it experiences the minute internal activities of the body.

There are several life forces at work in our body which provide energy to every part of it. When we have learnt to experience these forces in our body, we will be able to control their delicate movements also.

We are required to sit erect for practising *pranayama.* If we do not sit in an erect position, the spinal marrow gets disturbed which may cause harm. The chest, neck and head should be kept in a line. It will be difficult to do so in the beginning but after a few days of practice, it will become easy. Practice makes everything possible.

After sitting in a straight position you have to inhale and exhale in a rhythmic manner which means that the quantity of air which is drawn in should be the same as that which is forced out.

As you inhale and exhale, you may think of *Onkara* or any sacred name of the God you worship.

You have to concentrate entirely on your breathing. Slowly you will find that your body has become rhythmic and you feel as immensely fresh and energetic as you might never have experienced before.

Rigidity and dejection vanish, your face gradually acquires radiance and reflects the tranquillity that you have acquired in your mind. Your voice becomes sweet and persuasive having a touch of divinity.

To achieve all this will take some time. Soon you will be able to continue this practice while doing other chores. You will relish all types of activities whether you study, play, watch TV, and so on. You will achieve stability in your body and mind.

The regular practice of *pranayama* for a long time will divert the flow of energy upwards and help you to see nature in a new form. Do you know why all this is possible?

All this is possible because of the presence of *ida, pingala* and *sushumna* in your body. In fact, these channels exist in all living beings which possess a spinal cord.

Energy to the different parts of the body flow through the *ida* and the *pingala*, but when with the practice of *pranayama* the passage of *sushumna* opens, then the energy starts flowing upwards.

According to *yoga sastra* there are seven *chakras* (energy centres) existing in the *sushumna;* at the bottom of *sushumna* is the first centre *muladhara;* above it is the second one *svadhishthana;* then the third *manipura;* the fourth *anahata;* the fifth *vishudha,* the sixth *aagya,* and then the last *sahasradala padma.*

*Sahasradala padma* (a lotus with a thousand petals) centre resides in the top portion of the head. See the *chakras* in the following figure.

The whole energy starting from the *muladhara* (the lowest centre) moves upward till it reaches the highest centre, *sahasradala padma* which is yoga's ultimate objective.

According to *yoga sastra,* the most elevated form of energy in the human body is called *oja,* radiance, which is stored in the head. Some of your friends are more intelligent than you. For, the content of *oja* is more in their head. The one, who has less *oja* in him will be less intelligent.

Sometimes, some people's speech hold you mesmerised. This is also because of the great amount of *oja* in them.

*Oja* is present in all human beings. Yoga can increase the quantity of *oja.* The energy which stays in the *muladhara* is spent up in the form of sexual energy.

When with the help of yoga it is made to travel upwards, it gets transformed into *oja.* That is, the same energy gets converted into a number of different kinds of energies. All we need to do is to change its form.

This change can be effected by *pranayama.* Therefore, not only the *yoga sastra* but other religious scriptures also emphasize the need to follow *brahmacharya* (celibacy).

*Pranayama* also regulates the movement of the heart and keeps the lungs clear. Acidity is kept under control. Lifespan

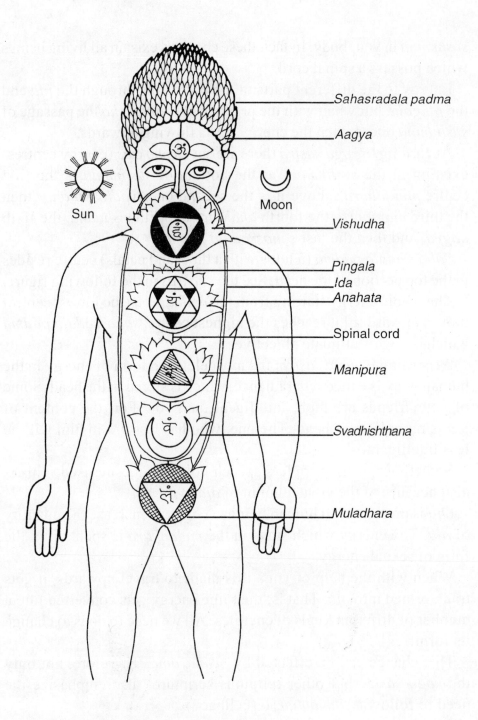

Kundalini

is increased. Your thoughts are not distracted and the power of concentration increases. You can do any work with interest.

*Pranayama* definitely increases the *oja* in us.

### Pratyahara

*Pratyahara* is made up of two words, *prati* and *ahara*. *Prati* means contrary and *ahara* means food.

*Savishayasamprayoge chittaswaroopanukar ivendriyanaam pratyaharah*

So *pratyahara* means sense organs behaving contrary to their food.

Do you know what the food of sense organs is? Their food is *vishaya* (worldly pleasures). For instance, the tongue wants to relish tasty food, the ears are eager to listen, the eyes remain in search of beauty, the nose loves to smell good, the skin loves the touch of things. The abstinence of these five sense organs from their normal pleasures is called *pratyahara*. It is practised after *pranayama*.

The attachment and detachment of the mind with the sense organs according to your requirement is *pratyahara*.

To experience external objects, sense organs, nerve centres of the brain, and mind are the three things required. Only when all three are connected with the outside object, can you experience that object.

Eyes, nose, tongue, ears and skin are the sense organs. With the help of the nerve centres of the brain these five sense organs carry out their work in the body. Then the mind plays its part. For instance, when the eyes work in accordance with the nerve centres of the brain, the mind too joins them and that is how we derive pleasure on seeing a beautiful object.

Sometimes you are asked by your mother to fetch some important articles from the market. On your way, you meet your friend. Instead of purchasing things, you start gossiping with your friend because you relish his talks more than doing your duty. Your mother is anxious at home and you are admonished when you reach home late.

This is due to a weak mind. It is the mind which allures you to indulge in such acts for which you repent later. Yoga emphasizes on the principle of self-help. In order to discipline our mind we should depend on ourselves and not on others.

By practising *pratyahara* we can control our mind and thereby increase our power. We can utilize these powers in useful activities.

A regular practice of yoga increases our efficiency in work.

Controlling the mind is indeed difficult. The mind is restless like an ape. Through the technique of *pratyahara* even the most restless mind can be brought under control.

How? You are required to sit silently and let your mind wander freely at its own sweet will. Let good and bad thoughts come to your mind. These thoughts will gradually vanish and you will become stable.

If you practise *pratyahara* daily with patience, you will find that lakhs of thoughts, which flood your mind, will gradually reduce to thousands and then to hundreds. This may take time, but regular practice will reduce the influx of thoughts. Slowly you will have control over the mind. Now it will not follow the sense organs at its will but only at your command.

Previously you used to act on the dictates of your mind like a mere slave. Now you will become its master and it will be your slave. Your mind will follow your command and act according to your wishes. You will then become perfect in performing *pratyahara*.

## Dharana

*Deshbandhashchittasya dharana*

(To control tendencies of the mind at a particular point is called *dharana*.)

When you practise *dharana* your mind will stay on a particular object for as long as you wish; thereafter, according to your wishes, will move to other objects.

For instance, you may focus on your heart and imagine the sky, a lotus

30

or ocean in your mind. As long as possible you may concentrate on this centre or you may concentrate on *sahasradala padma* dwelling in your head or on *aagya chakra* situated between the eyebrows.

You should practise this regularly. A particular characteristic of yoga is that even a little practice can produce good results.

### *Dhyana*

After *dharana* the mind is focused on *dhyana* (meditation).

*Tatra pratyay ekatanata dhyanam*

(When the mind is trained to concentrate on a particular object inside or outside the body, that state is called *dhyana*.)

During *dhyana* the mind is focused on one object only. You are required to sit straight during *dhyana* and close your eyes. In the beginning you should focus your mind on some solid object of your liking but gradually you can concentrate on something abstract.

The Divine Power is present in you. By meditating on that Power, you will feel it within you. This will enhance your mental power.

As compared to *dharana*, *dhyana* requires more concentration. During *dhyana* you detach yourself from your physical body and can see your real self.

You are ridden with many tensions—tension of getting through the examination, of securing first class or a good rank, tension of excelling in games, tension due to trifling matters, so on.

At this stage, *dhyana* comes to your rescue. *Dhyana* does not necessarily mean that you should concentrate on *aagya chakra* or on your heart only, but you can concentrate on any object.

You can perform all acts with full consciousness. You will then get the full benefits of *dhyana*. You will not get tensed because while eating and digesting the guava, your full attention is focused on it and nowhere else. Then your food will get digested properly because it will have all the digestive enzymes acting on it. This will lead you to good health. When you take food while being tense, formation of digestive enzymes stop and you cannot digest the food properly. Consequently, you are attacked by various diseases.

You may have seen vagabonds roaming without any direction. If you ask them to sit and attend to some work they will not be able to do so. However, if they conscientiously make a start, then they will be successful. Your mind is also like a vagabond, wandering aimlessly, but if you train your mind to concentrate on work it may give up the habit.

Sometimes, you keep your mind tense for no reason. You are not even aware of this tension which keeps your head restless with the result that it grows weaker day by day and your intellectual faculties diminish. When you sit in *dhyana* you let both your mind and body relax.

You will be able to experience the inhaling and exhaling process of your breathing. You will also be able to hear your heart beating.

### Samadhi

The stage of *samadhi* (meditation) comes after *dhyana*. *Samadhi* is the ultimate aim of yoga.

*Tadevarthamatranirbhrasam svaroopashunyamiv samadhih*
(When, while sitting in *dhyana* you become oblivious of yourself and the act of *dhyana* itself, that state is called *samadhi.*)

For attaining the stage of *samadhi* you need not depend on any object. Crossing the eight stages of yoga one by one, you can reach the ultimate stage, *samadhi,* for which you have to continue your practice regularly. This will, no doubt, take time. By practising yoga continuously with patience, you will steadily acquire proficiency. Even if you practise three methods (asana, *pranayama,* and *dhyana*), you will get full benefits of yoga. You will experience allround development of your personality.

*Samadhi* is not loss of consciousness, but achievement of transcendence, a state in which the mind, like a clear mirror reflects everything but is not clouded by anything.

32

## Conditions

Passing through the progressive stages, you should keep in mind a few points congenial to the process:

*Regularity and punctuality*: You have to practise yoga regularly. If you practise yoga for a few months and give up, you will have to start again from the very beginning. The regular practice of yoga will yield good results, and not doing it in fits and starts.

Punctuality is important. Yoga should be practised at a fixed time in the morning and evening after bath and in a happy state of mind.

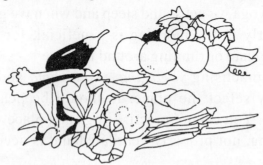

*Food*: Food should be taken four hours before or half an hour after the practice. It is not desirable to practise asana or *pranayama* immediately after eating. Food should be taken regularly and at a fixed time. Dinner should be taken at least four hours before going to sleep. This gives rest to the digestive organs while you sleep. Students should observe this rule strictly.

Food should preferably be vegetarian avoiding oily, spicy, heavy, fried and overcooked food. One should take nourishing food rather than care for taste only. Bananas and apples should be preferred to fried food items like *kachori* or samosa. Simple chapatis will be better than parathas or puris. Taking excessive spices harms the digestive system. Overcooking deprives the food of its nutritive value.

Healthy food consists of green vegetables, salads, fruits and milk. Meat should desirably be avoided. One should neither eat too much nor too little. A balance should be maintained.

*Clothes*: While practising yoga one should wear loose clothes in order to facilitate blood circulation. Tight clothes create obstructions in the movement of the body and could also be torn.

It is best to wear cotton clothes while practising yoga as they absorb the sweat and allow air into the body. Synthetic clothes cannot absorb sweat, and do not allow air to pass through. This is very harmful for the body, especially for the skin.

*Sleeping:* Anyone practising yoga should sleep early and get up early, preferably before sunrise, as getting up after sunrise is not conducive to health. After finishing the morning rituals, one should practise asana, *pranayama* and *dhyana.*

By practising yoga we get sound sleep and when we get up, we feel fresh. Rising early in the morning is beneficial, for it avoids the tension of getting late or running around in haste.

*Place*: While practising *yogasana, pranayama* and *dhyana* one should carefully select the place. It should be peaceful, clean, airy and solitary. You cannot practise yoga at a place which is very noisy, suffocating, not properly ventilated and is accessible to too many people.

It is equally advisable not to practise yoga at a place which is dirty, frightening and insecure because of hazards of fire or water and which is infested with insects or mosquitoes or has a danger of wild animals, snakes or scorpions. Practising yoga at such a place will affect your concentration. Therefore, practise yoga and *pranayama* at any beautiful and natural site which is safe or in any well-ventilated room.

Asana, *pranayama* and *dhyana* should be practised on a mattress or a blanket spread on the floor.

*Need for an expert guide*: *Yogasana* and *pranayama* should be practised under the guidance of an expert. After learning properly you can perform these yourself. In the beginning if you do not have the guidance of an expert, it would be harmful to you. Your nerves could be damaged or a bone could be displaced.

*The state of health*: You should not perform yoga if you are sick; or feel weakness after an illness; or if there is any problem in the spinal cord; or if you have undergone an operation recently.

If you are suffering from problems like diabetes or blood pressure and want to cure them through yoga, you should definitely practise it under the guidance of an expert, not otherwise.

*Company:* When you start practising yoga, you should be careful to stay away from undesirable or evil-minded persons. This is to prevent you from feeling uneasy or committing any wrong deeds.

Similarly, there are certain places which will perturb your mind whereas when you go to a temple or a church, you feel at peace with yourself.

This happens because of vibrations. Every place and every person reflects a particular kind of vibration. And your mind is conditioned according to the surrounding vibrations. Through the practise of yoga you will succeed in generating pure and peaceful vibrations. Thus, purify the atmosphere surrounding you.

*Physical limitations*: You should not overdo the asanas hoping to achieve early or quick results. You should try to bend your body as much as it allows you to do. You should sit in a particular asana for as long as you can easily do and take up only that asana in the beginning which you can perform without strain. It is harmful to use any kind of force on your body.

*Gradualism*: Gradual practice will make your body flexible and will enable you to perform even the most difficult asana. It is wrong to tire your body by doing many asanas for too long a period. Begin the practice for a short period and then go on increasing the duration of time gradually. This is the right way of doing asanas.

It is important to give rest to your body after performing an asana. Let your body relax.

Do not undertake any other form of exercise if you are practising yoga regularly.

**Personality Development**

The most important point to be kept in mind is that you should continue with your yoga practice without craving for results. Yoga

35

will certainly yield good results. To practise it with the desire of a reward is against the rules of yoga.

Yoga is the science of the human body as well as of the mind.

Good personality includes many things such as a balanced and healthy body; a good nature, patience, absence of anger, a calm mind, proficiency in work, games, studies, speech, dance and drama, and zeal and optimism.

Yoga helps to create energy in the body. If you meditate for an hour it will give you rest equivalent to what you can get by sleeping for several hours.

The practice of yoga helps in developing the qualities of creativity, concentration of mind and allround development.

At the mental level, yoga helps to control anger and to create noble feelings such as compassion and love in human beings.

At the intellectual level, yoga helps to develop the power of intellect, that is, the quality to discriminate between good and bad.

We have emphasized that the regular practice of asanas make your body healthy and well-balanced.

The practise of yoga will make your voice sweet and soft. If you are short-tempered, you will change into a polite person. You will find that everybody is happy with you.

Regular practice of yoga keeps laziness away, conserves human energy in the body which can be utilized properly whenever required. The practice of yoga increases efficiency and enables you to work more than otherwise.

When you increase your power of concentration, you can easily excel in studies, games, music, dance and speech, so on.

So yoga helps you to develop an ideal personality. Qualities of an ideal and developed personality are: a balanced and healthy body, optimism, patience, efficiency, developed memory, good knowledge, balanced behaviour and intellect, fearless and tensionless mind, capacity to take decisions and self-confidence.

A beautiful body is a natural gift but to keep it healthy and well-balanced depends upon our own efforts. The regular practice of yoga will help to keep our body well-balanced, healthy and active.

Obesity leads to various body ailments such as heart problem, high blood pressure, pain in the joints and panting just by doing a little physical work. The yogic exercises do not allow fat to accumulate in the body.

Many people suffer from weakness because of their frail body. Even if they wish, they cannot have food to their satisfaction. Owing to a weak digestive system, they are unable to digest the food and suffer from poor appetite.

The practice of yoga improves the digestive system. The enzymes are formed in sufficient quantity which help in digesting the food. This increases the appetite and removes physical debilities.

With regular practice of yoga, the body sweats sufficiently which keeps skin diseases away. Perspiration helps to purify blood. If the toxic matter is not expelled from the body by perspiration, it mixes with the blood and makes it impure causing many ailments. When the body perspires, it helps in purification of blood by throwing the waste matter out of the body and by increasing the count of white blood corpuscles (WBC) in the blood. After expulsion of toxic matter, the foul odour disappears from the body.

Some children do not grow tall. Here yoga comes to their help. If they practise *tadasana* they can increase their height. This way they can gain self-confidence.

A good health is a source of great joy. A sick man is a burden not only on others but also on himself. Regular practice of yoga will keep you healthy and you will participate in all the activities of life with joy and enthusiasm. To achieve this you will have to spare a little time daily.

A healthy body will serve you for your lifetime. The practice of asanas, *pranayama* and *dhyana* bring their rewards.

In case of certain incurable diseases where medical science has failed, the scientific method of yoga has come to the aid of patients. This is so because the body and the mind are closely related.

An interesting instance is the case of Amrita, who was a cancer patient. Govind used to tell her about yoga. While listening to him she realized that there was immense power in the soul which dwells in all of us. Amrita kept practising yoga regularly for a month. She felt a miraculous change in her body and mind. She felt very good and therefore she continued the practice. The white blood corpuscles in the body increased and the cancerous cells started diminishing. A feeling of immense solace came to her heart.

One day she went to the hospital for a check-up. After checking her, the doctors told her that she did not have any more symptoms of cancer in her body.

Amrita's family, hospital staff and her friends were delighted to hear her success.

Is this not a miracle of yoga?

(Amrita's case is quoted in *Yoga Sudha*, May 1999, published by the Vivekananda Centre, Bangalore.)

Many diseases can be cured through yoga. Yoga is a science.

### Panchakoshas

According to *yoga sastra*, the human body is not what is visible to us but consists of five fundamentals (bodies) called *panchakoshas*. *Taittiriya Upanishad* describes *panchakoshas.* They are:

*Annamaya kosha*: The physical body which is visible to us is the *annamaya kosha*. It is made of the food that we consume. It is the food which keeps the cells of the human body alive. Hence the name.

*Pranamaya kosha*: Our body has a maze of nerves through which the *prana* (life force) flows in the entire body. This is the *pranamaya kosha*. It is controlled by the *prana,* without which we will be lifeless.

*Manomaya kosha*: This consists of our mind and its position is higher than the physical body and the *prana.*

*Vigyanamaya kosha*: This is subtler than the mind. It is concerned with the intellect which is our discriminating power. It is superior to the physical body, *prana* and the mind. It is the intellect which decides what is good or bad for us.

*Anandamaya kosha*: This is concerned with the state of bliss—the ultimate goal of man. We develop a feeling of detachment towards the material objects of the world and get immersed in the Supreme Power.

A regular practice of yoga enables one to reach that stage.

The *koshas* make us understand how diseases originate in the human body.

Illnesses are of two kinds:

*Vyadhi:* This type of disease occurs owing to external conditions. You get malaria due to mosquito bite; or when you are attacked by germs present in the air, you fall sick, as in the case of a viral fever. Germs attack weak bodies.

A weak body has fewer number of white blood corpuscles which act as soldiers in the body. Whenever germs or virus of a particular disease attack the human body, these soldiers fight them.

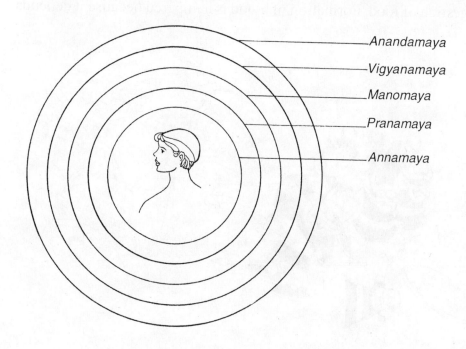

Panchakoshas

As stated earlier, a regular practice of yoga increases the number of white blood corpuscles and makes the body strong. Consequently, you will keep away from all sorts of diseases.

*Adhi:* The other kind of disease is known as *adhi*. This is caused when the mind is unbalanced, it loses its calmness and stability or is ridden with many worries, fears and tensions. When the mind is upset, symptoms of disease start appearing in the body. That is why such diseases are also called psychosomatic diseases.

Some of you may fall ill during the examination due to fear, worry and tension. While speaking on the stage you start trembling, your throat becomes dry and you feel giddy. When your mind loses balance, the *prana* also becomes unbalanced, which means that the breathing becomes irregular.

When the breathing process is disturbed, the nervous system loses its balance. Mental tension and irregular breathing also disturbs digestion of food. Formation of blood is hampered because it depends

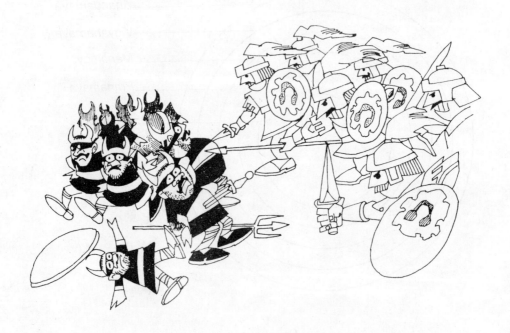

White Blood Corpuscles fighting germs

on the intake and digestion of our food. This results in making the body weak and vulnerable to attack by diseases.

These diseases are born in the *manomaya kosha* (mind).

We should treat all the three *koshas,* that is, *annamaya* (physical body), *pranamaya* (breathing process) and the *manomaya* to root out diseases. Yoga treats the patient at all the three levels.

To remove the disorders of the *annamaya kosha,* various asanas are performed. Some yogic techniques are also used for the internal cleansing of the body.

To remove disorders in the *pranamaya kosha,* balance must be brought back to the *nadis.* These *nadis* are so fine that they are not visible to the naked eye. It is visible in just one place in the whole body—the breathing centre.

If the flow of *prana shakti* is disturbed, the breathing region gets imbalanced too. Balance can be brought back by practising *pranayama.*

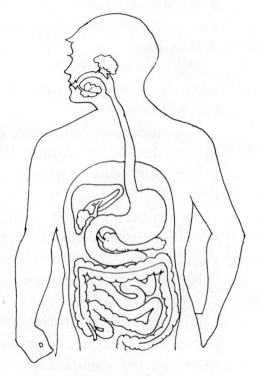

Digestive system

Owing to unnecessary and excessive exertion, worries on account of the future, competition, tension and fear, feelings of jealousy and enmity, etc. grow stronger and disturb the human mind with the result that diseases get an opportunity to afflict the body.

*Pranayama* makes the breathing process regular and rhythmic, removes mental tension, stops the mind from wandering and worrying. Mind becomes calm and stays in a blissful state. The digestive juices are formed in adequate quantity and blood formation continues regularly. The *urja* (energy) flows properly in the body and gradually the body becomes healthy. In this manner, disorders in the *manomaya kosha* are removed and the person becomes healthy.

*Suryanamaskara*: This particular yogic exercise is recommended for those persons who feel disappointed, frustrated and discouraged in life and also for those who feel physically and mentally tired and sick, suffer from lack of energy and irregular flow of blood to the heart. Regular practice of *suryanamaskara* will help them to get energy and new life from the sun. They will find a new zeal and hope in their life.

The sun rises everyday and brings energy, consciousness and new life to the world. The *suryanamaskara* is performed to draw more energy from the sun.

The whole body is benefited from the asanas. Muscles of the body become flexible and stiffness of joints disappear. Other ailments such as formation of gas, pain in the calves and swelling of veins are also removed.

Performing certain asanas contract and expand the digestive organs which in turn increase the appetite. These asanas also remove constipation, expel gas and increase digestive powers.

By the yogic method of treatment, every aspect of a disease is taken care of and rooted out completely.

In other systems of treatment, every aspect of a disease is not treated. With the help of medicines the disease is suppressed, with the result, *manomaya kosha* loses its balance and another *adhi* (disease) appears.

Performing certain *yogasanas* increase the circulation of blood and make it rush to the head. These asanas are the *sarvangasana, halasana, seershasana*, etc. Rapid circulation of blood in the head while performing the above mentioned exercises have a soothing effect on the nerves of the brain which help in removing mental tension and worries. You have sound sleep and you will feel fresh even if you sleep for a short time. You will also become more enthusiastic and active.

42

If asanas and *pranayama* are performed with concentration on different parts of the body, one can keep away from all types of diseases.

## Internal Cleaning

For cleaning the body internally, some methods have been recommended by yoga.

The *anunasika svasana* cleans the air passage; the *svana svasana* helps to rapidly expel the carbon dioxide from the body; the *mukhabhrastika* also performs the same function. By doing these exercises, the quantity of oxygen which is so essential for life increases in the body.

The mind feels joy, the body becomes more active and the feelings of tiredness and uneasiness are driven away.

The *kapalabhati* expels the carbon dioxide from the blood, makes the cells of the head active and sharpens the intellect.

The *neti* purifies the organs of the head and neck, as well as the air passage. It also helps in curing sinusitis.

The *dhauti* purifies all organs from the cavity of the mouth to the stomach. It removes digestive disorders.

The *nauli* activates various digestive organs in the body and helps to bring forth digestive juices to mix with the eaten food.

By following the method of *trataka* one can remove defects in the eye-sight. Even those who use spectacles can give up using them if they regularly practice *trataka*.

The *sankha prakshalana* method cleans the intestines, which keeps away laziness and makes the body active.

*Pranayama* is an integral part of yoga. It enables the respiratory system to function properly and rhythmically.

You get rid of chronic cough and cold, headache and can also avoid heart diseases.

Acidity and other stomach disorders can be kept at bay. People with high or low blood pressure can also get relief.

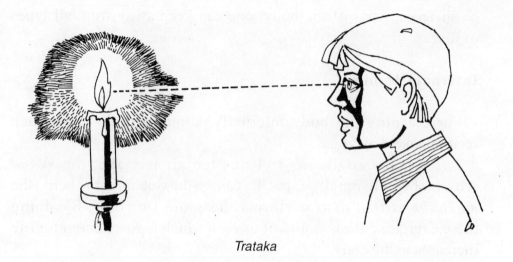

*Trataka*

As the asanas are performed, the respiration is rhythmic which expels carbon dioxide from the lungs and takes in oxygen. Deep breathing makes the lungs strong and prevents all diseases relating to respiration.

## In Old Age

The regular practice of yoga removes tiredness of body and mind. Age is prolonged.

As age increases, the strength of the body decreases. The human body is made of cells. During childhood and young age, new cells continue to form in the body. This process continues even when the old cells are dying.

When old age begins, the formation of new cells slows down and gradually stops completely.

With yoga, the process of formation of new cells goes on continuously. Even with the increase in age the body does not weaken and symptoms of old age do not appear. A yogi stays young both in physical and mental ability.

44

A yogi, who is much advanced in age may look quite young. His voice is sweet, soft, effective and haunting. You feel that there is a strange, spiritual aura surrounding them. This is the magic of yoga.

Actually a man becomes old not due to age but due to the condition of his body. The practice of yoga enables you to keep your body young. To have a good personality, you must keep away from laziness which is actually responsible for many of your failures.

*Yogasanas* remove laziness. Yoga coupled with light food, makes the body active and smart. By practising yoga you can increase your efficiency in work.

The scientific technique of yoga is based on the principle that in normal condition, muscles of the body should remain at complete rest so that energy is not wasted. They should remain soft like a flower but, when required, should become as strong as steel.

What usually happens is that even while resting we keep our body tense and do not allow it to relax. There is really no need to do that but we behave so owing to our habit and waste our energy. Consequently, when we require energy for doing a certain work, we do not have enough left with us.

When we do not need to use our body we still keep it tense, and we expend our energy. When we start working we do not have enough energy.

When we do *yogasana*, the muscles of the body are stretched and then allowed to relax. This is repeated over and again. By doing so the muscles become soft and the body is free from tension. In *yogasanas,* the body is pulled out of a stupor to a state of activity and movement which generates *urja* (energy). Thereafter, the body is allowed to rest which is a state of non-movement. In this way, the energy is stored in the body and can be put to use when required.

No other system of physical exercises can conserve energy in this manner. You may be thinking that aerobics, exercises, dance and sports, can also keep the body healthy, but only to an extent.

Yoga removes the weaknesses of head and improves the intellect, memory and power of concentration.

## Concentration

It often happens that you are not aware of what type of shops there are on your regular route to school. There may be a tailor's shop on the way but when you return home and your mother asks you whether the shop was open, you are not able to give correct information to her.

Lack of awareness is the main reason for your failure. If you possess the quality of awareness, then you can achieve many a success in your life. How can you acquire this quality?

The practice of yoga can help you acquire awareness.

When you perform asanas you first concentrate on your body and then on your mind. The mind acquires the habit of being alert. By awakening your mind by regular practice, you will gradually attend to your daily chores with full awareness and concentration.

If your mind is attentive, you will always have presence of mind.

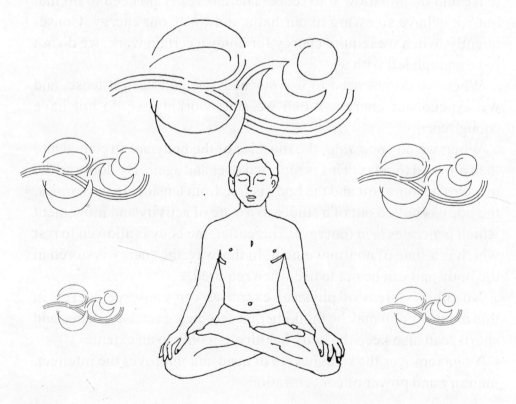

Wherever you live, you will always be conscious of what is happening around you.

When you attempt *yogasanas* you have to focus your mind on one point, which enhances your power of concentration and awareness. Various exercises such as *suryanamaskara, halasana, seershasana, chakrasana, kapalabhati* (purification of the alimentary canal), *pranayama* and so on increase the flow of blood to the head, improving your intellectual power as well as memory. There is a soothing effect on the nerves which helps in removing your feelings of tension, irritation, worry and lack of sleep. By enjoying a good sleep your brain has full rest and when you wake up, you feel fresh. You can concentrate only when you feel fresh.

Concentration is very important for education and acquiring knowledge. Whether the education is of an ordinary or specialized nature, you cannot achieve anything without concentration. The more the concentration, the better is the quality of work.

Success in any field of human activity depends on the power of concentration. Proficiency in the field of art, literature or music can be acquired only by single-minded devotion and practice.

*Dhyana* is one of the methods of yoga which is used for practising concentration.


**Memory Training**

You learn and memorize lessons very well, but at the time of test, forget answers to the questions and even with your best efforts cannot recollect them with the result that you fare badly in the test. You are very upset.

The first requirement for mental development is a good memory. You may read and learn a great deal but if you do not remember these when required, then you will not be able to use what you have learnt.

*Yogasanas* such as *halasana, seershasana, sarvangasana* and the technique of *kapalabhati* improve the blood circulation in the head, rectify defects in the brain and improve the memory.

*Pranayama* and *dhyana* help to become clear-headed. They also increase your power of concentration and improve memory.

The regular practice of yoga promotes development of intellectual faculties such as intelligence, concentration and reasoning, and memory.

Swami Vivekananda said that knowledge exists inside man. It does not come from outside. What we get from outside is experience and information. Even that is already there in man.

Isaac Newton discovered the law of gravity. It came out of him effortlessly.

Swami Vivekananda believed that every human being is gifted with a treasure of knowledge. A regular practice of yoga uncovers it.

Regular yoga practice helps to balance the emotions such as love and anger. One also gets rid of mental struggle between good and evil. The practice of asanas inculcates the quality of patience in you. It also creates awakening in you and helps you to keep away from disappointments and tensions.

Our five enemies, namely, *kama, krodha, mada, moha* and *lobha* reside in us.

*Kama* means desire. *Krodha* means anger. You know very well how harmful anger is for us. *Mada* means ego, false pride. *Lobha* means greed which can lead a man to commit any crime. You can destroy these enemies by following the path of yoga. *Moha* means desire or attachment.


**Self-control**

Often you are not in a mood to do any work. Do you know what mood is? It is actually the mind. You lag behind owing to your mind. It is the mind which does not allow you to work or study.

The science of yoga can guide one on how to stop the mind from wandering with no goal or get involved in useless matters and instead acquire the quality of concentration. It becomes easy for us to shift it from one subject to another.

As you might have experienced, you are able to understand a subject such as geography or physics very thoroughly even if it is very difficult, because you find it interesting. On the other hand, some other subject such as history or mathematics may not interest you even if it is easy to understand. The reason is that you do not study that subject with full concentration. Yoga will enable you to study any subject with interest and understand it.

You will find that you can easily concentrate on one subject and

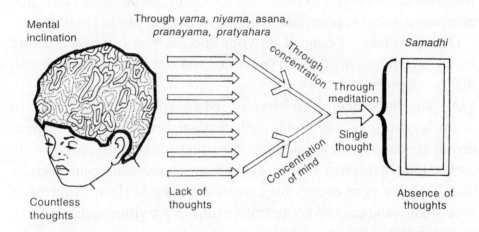

Controlling the mind through yoga

then on another. You will not think of the past or future events but focus your mind on the present. This will enable you to pay full attention to any work and complete it successfully. Yoga calms the disturbed mind and disciplines it.

The basic nature of mind is its fickleness. The mind contains countless thoughts. These thoughts are reduced by practising *yama, niyama,* asana, *pranayama* and *pratyahara.* With the practice of *dhyana* thoughts are concentrated on one subject.

*Dhyana* reduces the number of thoughts to only one. The state of *samadhi* leads to voidness and complete absence of thoughts.

49

In this way, fickleness of mind disappears and it becomes stable and peaceful. More, your behaviour and thinking are balanced and your speech is well-controlled.

Balanced behaviour is the quality of a seasoned person. He does not get agitated for any reason. People with balanced behaviour leave good impression on others.

A cultured and disciplined person should control anger, irritation, tension over trifling matters and worries.

One should cultivate a poised behaviour with the help of yoga.

A person who has a balanced thinking does not feel disturbed or worried in adverse circumstances but, by remaining calm and composed, takes appropriate decisions. He does not act in haste.

Owing to lack of control on your speech, you often say absurd things. You have something in your mind and you speak out in a manner that is not proper.

As you have been told already, when you reach the stage of *pratyahara* in yoga, you avoid worthless thoughts. When such thoughts do not appear in your mind, there is no question of your indulging in useless talk. In this way you can avoid many unnecessary controversies and thus save your energy for constructive work, show progress in your studies and can use your creative time in activities such as sports, dance, music, writing and delivering speeches.

Yoga is indeed a preparation for physical strength and building up our mental resources. The two together create balanced outlook.

## Compatibility

Sometimes you get irritated over small matters, feel lonely, you are disappointed and live in isolation. The reason is the lack of compatibility, cooperation and adjustment with others.

The problem can be solved by yoga. Yoga increases your efficiency and enables you not only to attend to your own work but also to others' problems.

When you help others by doing their work, they will be happy with you and you will also have a rare feeling of happiness and satisfaction.

The yogic style of life lays emphasis on selfless service. It motivates you not to expect any reward from anybody in return of any favour done to him. If you follow this principle, there is no possibility of your involvement in tension.

The wall of misunderstanding between you and others will vanish. In this way, you will develop compatibility with all, which is an important characteristic of a wise person. The principles enunciated in the *yoga sastra* really help in developing human personality.

## Value Of Patience

Patience or *kshama* or forbearance has been a value which India's culture has fostered and cherished. *Kshama* is *balam* (strength) of the weak and a glory or embellishment for the strong.

Asanas are performed in a slow and steady manner. The slow process of asanas will ingrain the quality of patience in you.

It has a great significance for an integrated personality. You must have noticed that a goldsmith fashions beautiful ornaments by working patiently. Artists practise for years on end to achieve perfection in their work.

Patience breeds humility. Patience is the ornament of man.

You can develop patience in you with the regular practice of *yogasana*. When you practice yoga regularly, instead of behaving like an escapist, you will grapple with your problems in a reposed manner. You will keep working on your problems steadily till you have solved them. You will be able to sit calmly till you have learnt your lesson.

You will have sufficient physical strength to sit at a place for a long period. Moreover, you will be able to apply your mind to the work you have taken up till it is completed.

Many children get frightened before taking part in competitions concerning sports, debates and speeches. You must have said, 'Yes, I am afraid.'

You may fear that you may forget the lesson you have memorized in the examination. Or what will happen if your friends do not turn up on your birthday!

The technique of yoga can help you overcome your fears. Three important channels exist in our body. They are the *ida*, *pingala* and *sushumna*. The *ida* represents negative and the *pingala* positive character, while the *sushumna* acts as a balancing factor.

In yoga, the process of *pranayama* activates the *sushumna* channel, which removes baseless fears and worries in your mind and instils in it a unique feeling of self-confidence.

Yoga helps to develop an optimistic attitude in your mind and removes useless worries. Whenever you face a problem, you think of solving it and do not waste time and energy by being puzzled over it. You become bold and face problems with a positive mind.

In fact, fear does not enter our body from outside but is born inside.

## No Mental Conflicts

At the emotional level, yoga redeems you from mental conflicts. Perhaps you do not know the meaning of mental conflict, even though you usually experience it. You are often in a fix whether you should study or watch a good film on television, which is what is meant by mental conflict.

With the practice of yoga, this type of mental struggle disappears.

Yoga helps to awaken your intellectual faculties. You are then able to decide for yourself what is good for you and you follow that.

With regular exercise of yoga you will find as much pleasure in studies as you will find in watching a film. Even more.

Usually you suffer from lack of ability to take decisions yourself about what you will do, what direction you will follow, what subjects you will take and how you will begin your career. For small matters you depend upon decisions taken by others.

52

The regular use of yoga builds self-confidence in you. You may consult others but you will decide for yourself what is right and what is wrong for you.

Yoga helps you to develop the capacity to take correct decisions.

## Spiritual Growth

Do you know that we are what we think? If you think in the negative and consider yourself weak, you will definitely become that. The practice of yoga awakens in man a consciousness that he is a part of the supreme power. He feels strong and competent.

During *pranayama* when we exhale, we should imagine that we are throwing out all the debilities from our body. When we inhale, we should imagine that the supreme power is entering our heart and body.

During meditation when we think of the radiant sun, the bottomless and boundless ocean, and the high mountains, it makes us realize that we are also a part of them.

These techniques of yoga enhance our mental strength and self-esteem. Self-confidence is the most important part of a man's personality.

On the one hand, yoga develops concentration of mind, memory, intellectual faculty, self-confidence and will power, on the other it keeps away all distractions of mind by enhancing inner strength in man and by awakening consciousness in him.

The practice of yoga not only removes depression and worries in you, but also gives you hope. The techniques of yoga such as *pranayama, pratyahara, dhyana* make you realize that the truth exists within you. The realization of truth gives you the feeling of deep satisfaction irrespective of success or failure. This feeling removes disappointment and instils hope in you.

Yoga is a means of self-realization. It awakens in us the feeling that all living beings have the same supreme power pervading in them. This awakens the feeling of universal love in us.

Selfless action accelerates spiritual development in us. It is through spiritual development that we can act selflessly while living in this world.

*Yoga sastra* tells us that real happiness lies within us and we can realize it through the technique of *dhyana*. Yoga is an integral aspect of the spiritual journey. The confidence it gives and the calm of mind it creates are essential for spiritual growth.

## One Earth, One Family

*Vasudhaiva kutumbakam* (the whole universe is my family) is the message of our ancient culture.

It is our country, which for the first time gave this message to the world. The basic principle of our culture is harmony which means feelings of equality and brotherhood. In spite of the fact that we possess a glorious cultural tradition, we find that destructive forces have become strong as a result of which we witness violence, tension and turbulence.

All this adversely affects the progress of not only our country but that of the whole world. Owing to the pursuance of narrow self-interests, the entire world is proceeding towards destruction.

It is sad that we blame one another for it.

We are the foundation on which rests the progress of the world. Therefore, the responsibility of saving humanity from destruction also lies on our shoulders.

Yoga corrects imbalance in human behaviour. Yoga awakens consciousness in human beings which enables us to see humanity as one.

Yoga creates awareness in human beings that they all have the same soul within them. This awareness will elevate them above their narrow self-interests. They will develop love for the entire mankind, which has been our cultural goal—one earth, one family. This ideal lifts us above the narrow circle of religion, caste, language and community to realize the dream of *vasudhaiva kutumbakam*.

54

You have understood how *yoga sastra* has the capacity to develop human personality at all levels—physical, mental, emotional and spiritual. What you actually need is to understand yoga, learn it and make it a part of your life through practice.

Our body is like a splendid palace which is matchless in its form and function. It is important that it is looked after well regularly. Only by remaining healthy will it be able to attend to its daily chores and also other works essential for our development and for humanity's wellbeing.

You can achieve peace of mind by practising yoga. No other form of physical exercise lays emphasis on the control of mind and mental tranquillity as does yoga. That is why it is considered a supreme science. The science of yoga creates self-discipline in man.

Mind has immense energy but we do not know how to preserve it. For reason of our fickle-minded nature, our energy gets wasted. When it is made still by practising *dhyana* and is focused on a particular point and is at peace, it can be useful.

By practising yoga, our mind will become so powerful that even when we are surrounded by bad thoughts none of them can enter our mind. This mental strength is essential to achieve full development of personality.

You may have observed that some persons possess many good qualities such as courage, self-confidence, patience, capacity to work hard and sharp intellect. You are also impressed by these qualities.

The fact is that we all possess these qualities but they are lying dormant. The practice of yoga can awaken these qualities and we can realize their presence within us. We will be surprised to find the positive change in us.

The yogic technique of *dhyana* will enable us to detach ourselves from the external world and turn inwards to realize our soul which is a part of the Absolute. We will also experience wonderful bliss. To achieve this, we have to control our mind by practising yoga regularly.

You know that the seed is hidden inside the fruit. We have to put the seed in the soil and feed the soil with manure, water, air and sun. Only then there appears a sprout which turns into a plant and then becomes a fruit-bearing tree. Similarly, with the practice of yoga, our mind becomes calm and free of tension which enables the energy lying latent within us to come out.

The bliss which is the boon of yoga is not affected by any sorrow or joy of the external world but flows within us like a spring, and also overwhelming like an ocean. Spreading like a cloud, it rains and drenches one and all in its divine nectar.

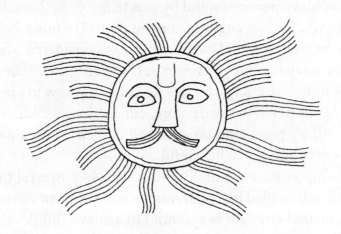